Running Log

Roger Hollis

Published 2017 by HumorOutcasts Press
Printed in the United States of America

ISBN: 0-9994127-1-X
ISBN-13: 978-0-9994127-1-8

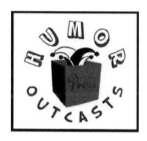

**Whatever your goals,
this log will help keep
you
motivated to reach them
(and give you a
little chuckle at the
same time)**

Roger Hollis

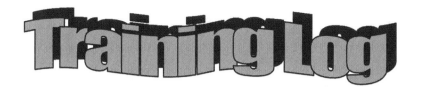

by Roger Hollis

This training log belongs to:

_____

And is a training log

from:

_____

to:

_____

Whether you're a beginner, a long time runner, run just for fun and exercise or are an ardent racer, we all have a variety of "tools" we use to keep us motivated.

One of my long time "tools" is a training log. I've got dozens that I have filled in over the years. I still keep them (I'm not sure I know why?)

They are my guides to tracking the miles I log to reach my annual goal.

While this training log provides you with a weekly summary of your progress, I've added a little whimsy for each week in the form of a cartoon to perhaps keep you motivated but also, hopefully, to add a small chuckle to your day.

Enjoy

Roger Hollis

" *Motivation is what gets you started, habit is what keeps you going*"

"*I'm not addicted to running, I can quite as soon as I finish one more race*"

"*You don't have to go fast, you just have to go*"

"*Runner's highs don't last but neither does bathing, that's why running daily is recommended*"

"*You know you're a runner when you come home exhausted and then go for a 5 mile run*"

" *The urgent need to go will occur at the furthest point from the Port-A-Potty*"

"*No one ever drowned in sweat*"

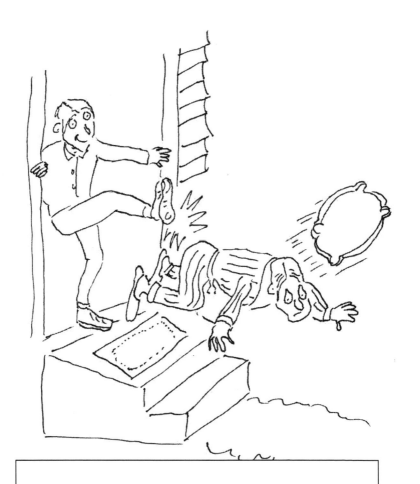

**<u>Get
back
out
there!</u>**

MONTH			COURSE	NOTES: temp, wind, pace etc.
day	distance	time		
		TOTAL		
WEEK				
last wk ytd		TOTAL		
YTD				

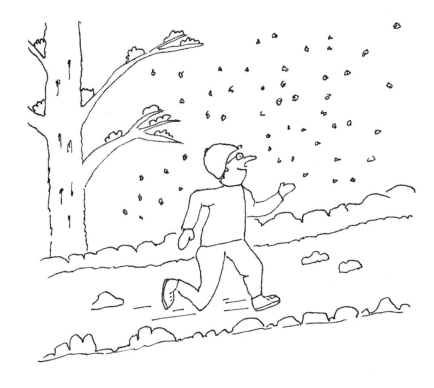

**If it's "too cold"**
**for a run you're**
**obviously not a**
**runner**

MONTH _____

day	distance	time	COURSE	NOTES: temp, wind, pace etc.
WEEK		**TOTAL**		
last wk ytd				
YTD		**TOTAL**		

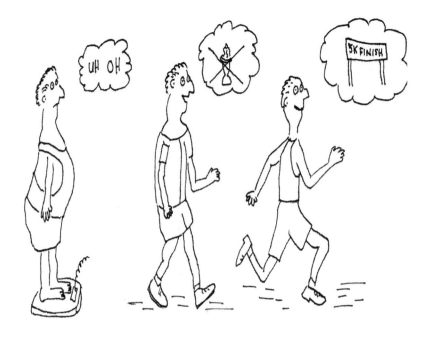

<u>*If it's going to be,*</u>
<u>*it starts*</u>
<u>*with me*</u>

MONTH			COURSE	NOTES: temp, wind, pace etc.
day	distance	time		
WEEK		TOTAL		
last wk ytd				
YTD		TOTAL		

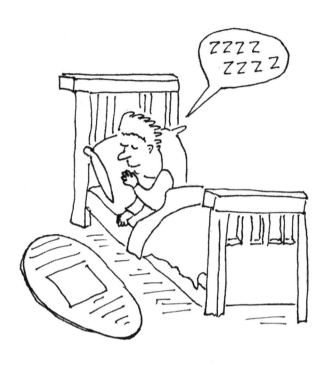

You'll get a lot more compliments for working out than you will for sleeping in.

MONTH ___			COURSE	NOTES: temp, wind, pace etc.
day	distance	time		
WEEK		**TOTAL**		
last wk ytd				
YTD		**TOTAL**		

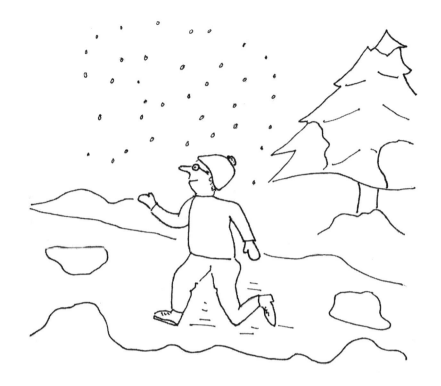

**It's only cold if you're standing still!**

MONTH ___

day	distance	time	COURSE	NOTES: temp, wind, pace etc.

WEEK ___ TOTAL

last wk ytd

YTD TOTAL

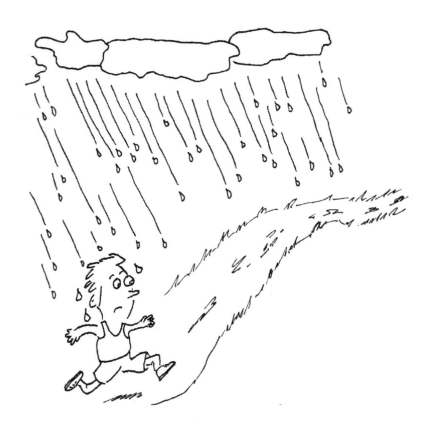

Running in the rain:
Exercise, therapy and a shower all at the same time

MONTH

day	distance	time	COURSE	NOTES: temp, wind, pace etc.

WEEK		TOTAL		
last wk ytd				
YTD		TOTAL		

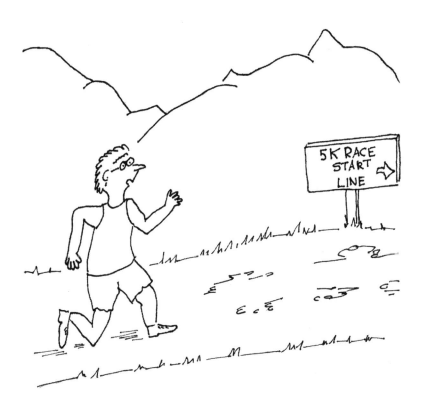

If you're looking for a sign, this is it.

MONTH ___			COURSE	NOTES: temp, wind, pace etc.
day	distance	time		
		TOTAL		
WEEK ___				
last wk ytd				
YTD		TOTAL		

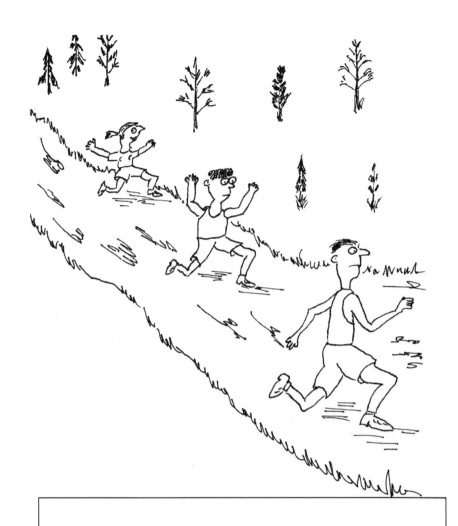

You don't have to be a fit in order to get fit

MONTH

day	distance	time	COURSE	NOTES: temp, wind, pace etc.
WEEK		TOTAL		
last wk ytd				
YTD		TOTAL		

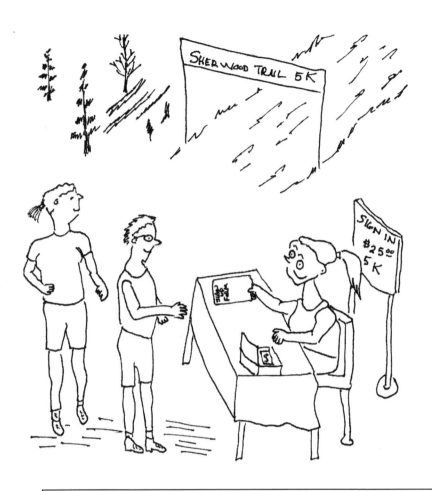

You know you're a runner when you pay to run in a race on the trail you run for free any other time.

MONTH			COURSE	NOTES: temp, wind, pace etc.
day	distance	time		
WEEK		TOTAL		
last wk ytd				
YTD		TOTAL		

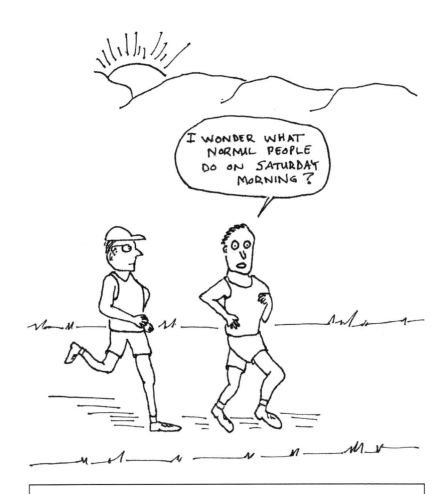

You know you're a runner when you ask this question.

MONTH			COURSE	NOTES: temp, wind, pace etc.
day	distance	time		
WEEK		TOTAL		
last wk ytd				
YTD		TOTAL		

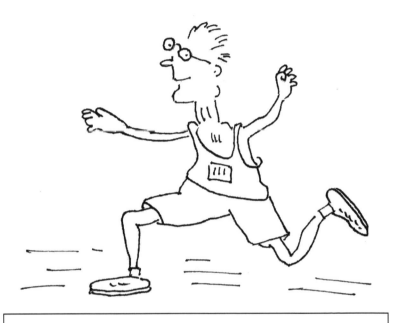

The older I get, the more value I get out of my running fee!

MONTH___			COURSE	NOTES: temp, wind, pace etc.
day	distance	time		
WEEK		TOTAL		
last wk ytd				
YTD		TOTAL		

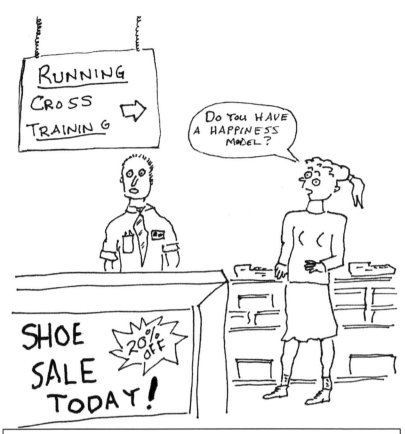

You can't buy hap-
piness but you can
buy new running
shoes and that's
kind of like the
same thing.

MONTH			COURSE	NOTES: temp, wind, pace etc.
day	distance	time		
	WEEK	TOTAL		
	last wk ytd			
	YTD	TOTAL		

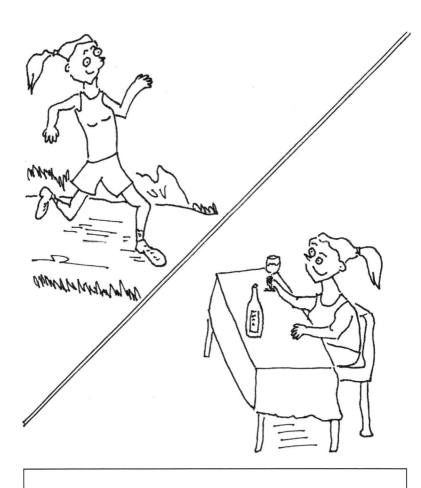

Run now.

Wine later.

MONTH____			COURSE	NOTES: temp, wind, pace etc.
day	distance	time		
WEEK		TOTAL		
last wk ytd				
YTD		TOTAL		

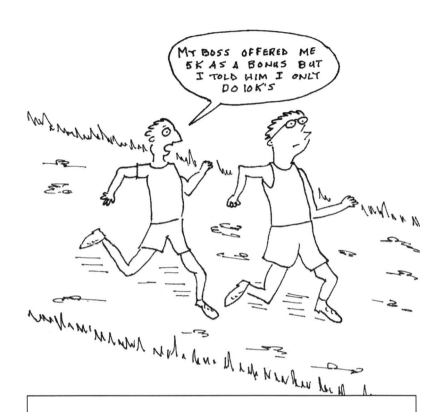

If 5K means 3.1 miles, not $5,000, then you're a runner.

MONTH___			COURSE	NOTES: temp, wind, pace etc.
day	distance	time		
WEEK___		TOTAL		
last wk ytd				
YTD		TOTAL		

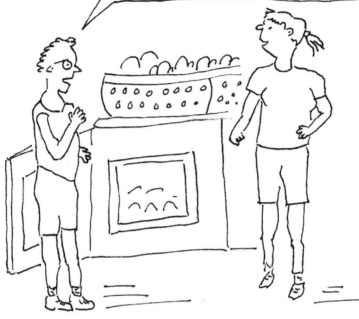

You know you're a runner when 90% of your laundry is running attire!

MONTH			COURSE	NOTES: temp, wind, pace etc.
day	distance	time		
WEEK		TOTAL		
last wk ytd				
YTD		TOTAL		

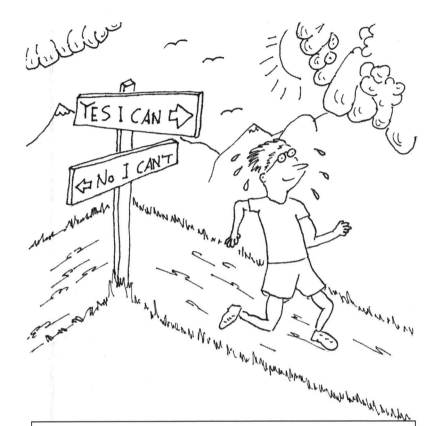

Success comes in cans, failure in can'ts.

MONTH____			COURSE	NOTES: temp, wind, pace etc.
day	distance	time		
WEEK____		TOTAL		
last wk ytd				
YTD		TOTAL		

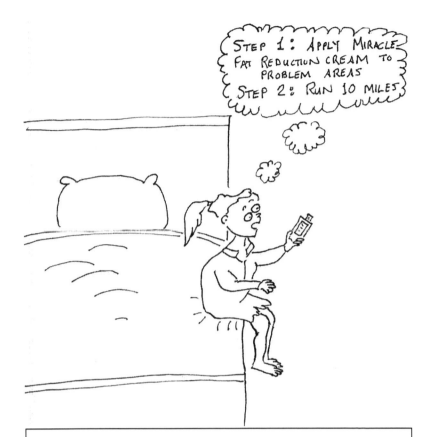

You don't get what you wish for, you get what you work for.

MONTH			COURSE	NOTES: temp, wind, pace etc.
day	distance	time		
		TOTAL		
WEEK				
last wk ytd				
YTD		TOTAL		

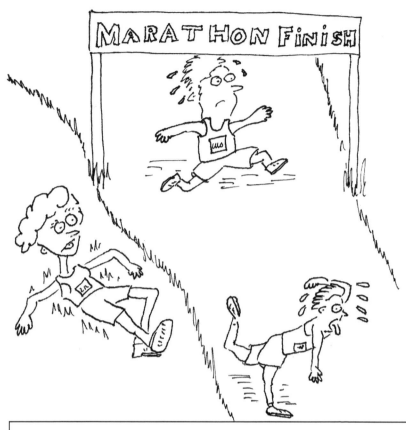

You have to forget your last marathon before signing up for another.
Your mind can't know what's coming

MONTH ___

day	distance	time	COURSE	NOTES: temp, wind, pace etc.

WEEK		TOTAL
last wk ytd		
YTD		TOTAL

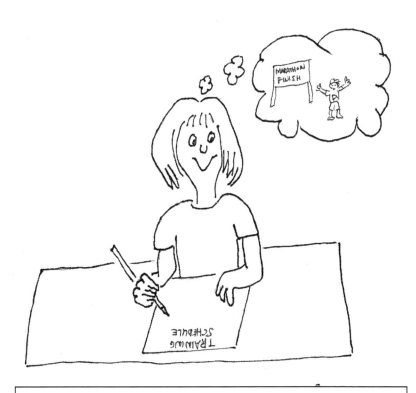

Have a dream, make a plan, go for it!

MONTH___			COURSE	NOTES: temp, wind, pace etc.
day	distance	time		
		WEEK TOTAL		
		last wk ytd		
		YTD TOTAL		

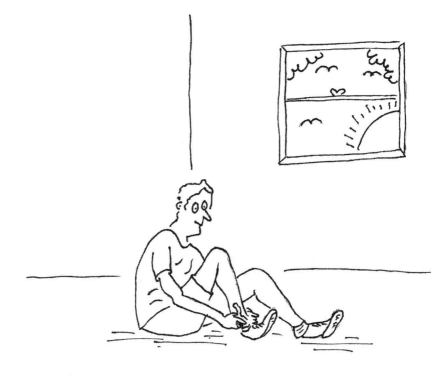

<u>Life is not a spectator sport, lace up your shoes and go for a run.</u>

MONTH ___

day	distance	time	COURSE	NOTES: temp, wind, pace etc.

WEEK ___		TOTAL
last wk ytd		
YTD		TOTAL

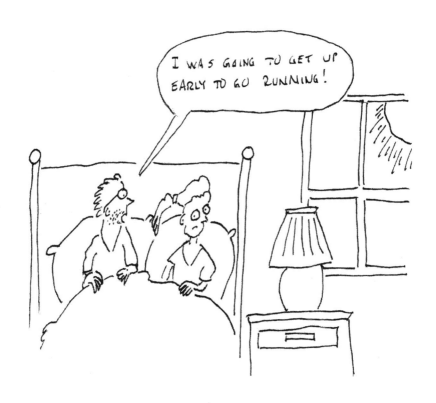

Actions speak louder than words. That's the reason you go for a run instead of talking about going for a run

MONTH

day	distance	time	COURSE	NOTES: temp, wind, pace etc.
WEEK		TOTAL		
last wk ytd				
YTD		TOTAL		

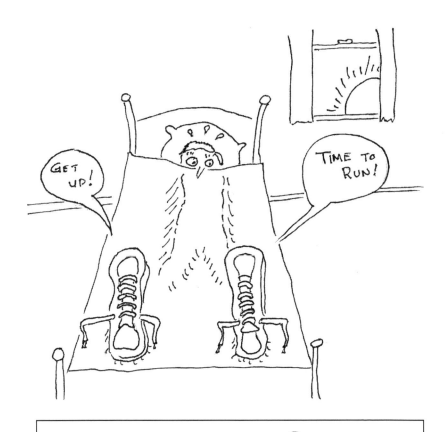

30 min a day, 5 days a week = 2.5 hrs out of 168 hours = 1.5 % a week.
NO EXCUSES

MONTH			COURSE	NOTES: temp, wind, pace etc.
day	distance	time		
WEEK		TOTAL		
last wk ytd				
YTD		TOTAL		

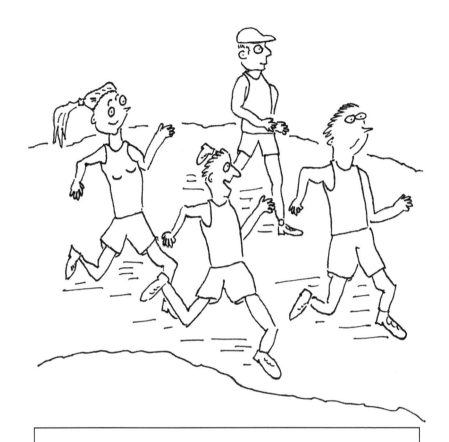

Group runs, better than group therapy

MONTH___			COURSE	NOTES: temp, wind, pace etc.
day	distance	time		
WEEK___		TOTAL		
last wk ytd				
YTD		TOTAL		

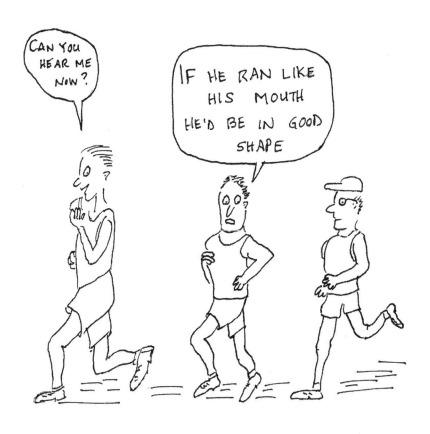

Remember, only you can prevent flabbiness!

MONTH ___

day	distance	time	COURSE	NOTES: temp, wind, pace etc.

WEEK ___ TOTAL

last wk ytd

YTD TOTAL

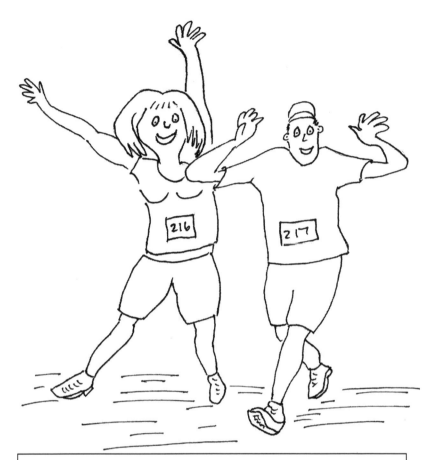

The moment when you see your friends with a camera at the race.

MONTH			COURSE	NOTES: temp, wind, pace etc.
day	distance	time		
WEEK		TOTAL		
last wk ytd				
YTD		TOTAL		

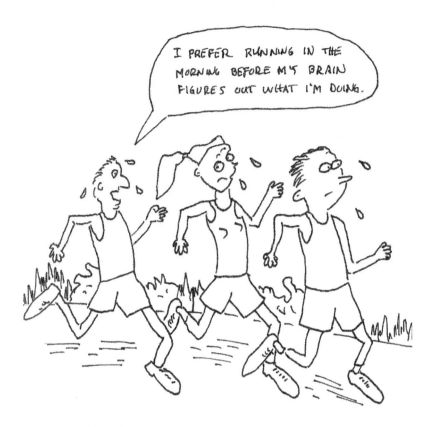

Running is 70% physical, 20% mental, 10% crazy or have I got that backwards?

MONTH _____

day	distance	time	COURSE	NOTES: temp, wind, pace etc.

WEEK	TOTAL
last wk ytd	

YTD	TOTAL

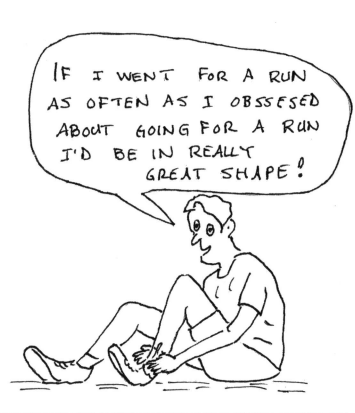

The hardest thing
for runners is
getting dressed.
After that you're
committed

MONTH _____

day	distance	time	COURSE	NOTES: temp, wind, pace etc.
WEEK		**TOTAL**		
last wk ytd				
YTD		**TOTAL**		

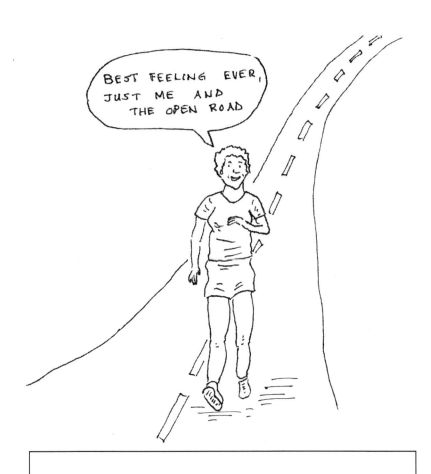

You will want to
stop.

DON'T

MONTH ____

day	distance	time	COURSE	NOTES: temp, wind, pace etc.

WEEK		TOTAL
last wk ytd		
YTD		TOTAL

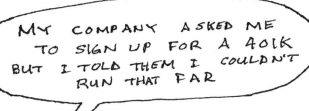

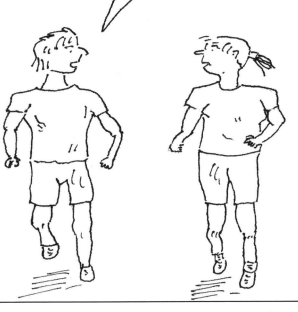

Discipline is doing what you don't want to do so you can do what you really want to do.

MONTH ____			COURSE	NOTES: temp, wind, pace etc.
day	distance	time		
WEEK		TOTAL		
last wk ytd				
YTD		TOTAL		

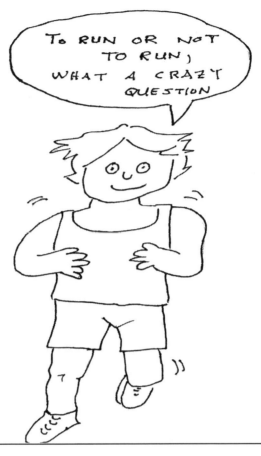

Log out

Shut down

Go run

MONTH___			COURSE	NOTES: temp, wind, pace etc.
day	distance	time		
WEEK		TOTAL		
last wk ytd				
YTD		TOTAL		

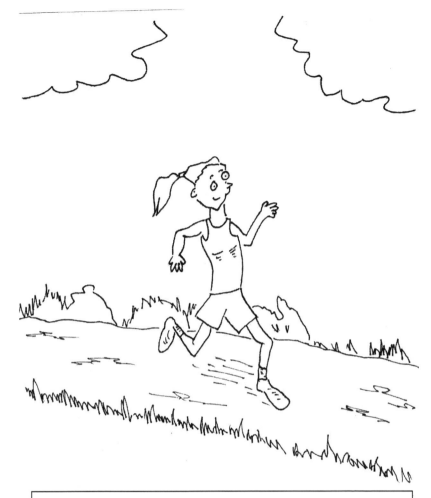

Think about how far you have gone, not about how far you have to go.

MONTH _____

day	distance	time	COURSE	NOTES: temp, wind, pace etc.

WEEK		TOTAL
last wk ytd		
YTD		**TOTAL**

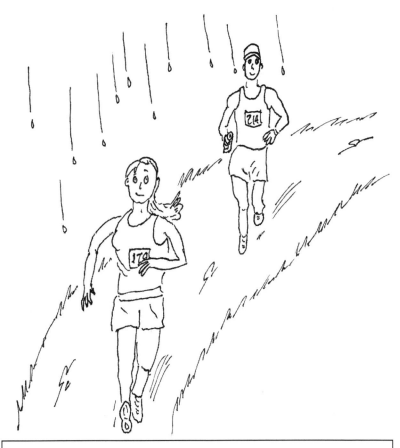

**You know you're a runner when someone asks you "what happens when it rains" and you laughingly say "you get wet"**

MONTH____			COURSE	NOTES: temp, wind, pace etc.
day	distance	time		
WEEK		TOTAL		
last wk ytd				
YTD		TOTAL		

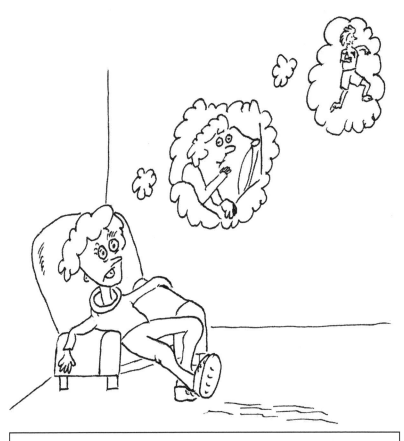

When you feel like crap, don't take a nap. Go for a run, you'll feel good when it's done!

MONTH			COURSE	NOTES: temp, wind, pace etc.
day	distance	time		
WEEK		TOTAL		
last wk ytd				
YTD		TOTAL		

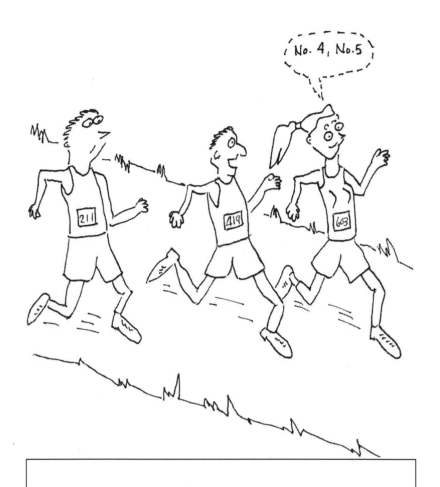

It's rude to count people as you pass them
(out loud)

MONTH				COURSE	NOTES: temp, wind, pace etc.
day	distance	time			
WEEK		TOTAL			
last wk ytd					
YTD		TOTAL			

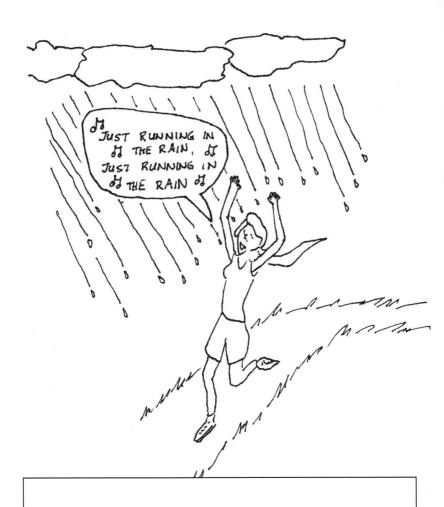

Best time to run?
55 degrees and a
light drizzle!

MONTH _____

day	distance	time	COURSE	NOTES: temp, wind, pace etc.

WEEK		TOTAL
last wk ytd		
YTD		TOTAL

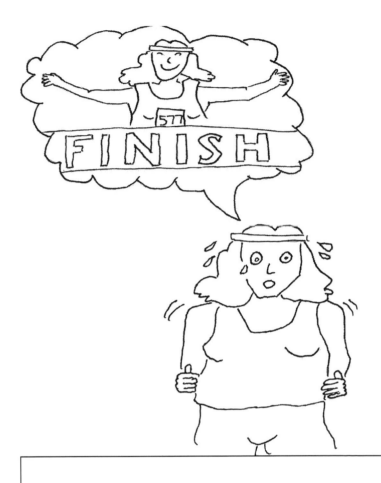

Dreams don't work unless you do.

MONTH _____

day	distance	time	COURSE	NOTES: temp, wind, pace etc.

WEEK		TOTAL
last wk ytd		
YTD		TOTAL

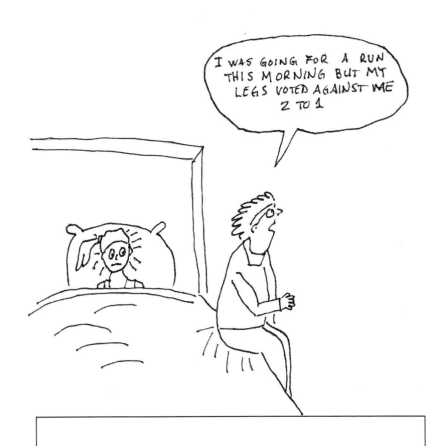

Discipline creates performance.

MONTH			COURSE	NOTES: temp, wind, pace etc.
day	distance	time		
WEEK		TOTAL		
last wk ytd				
YTD		TOTAL		

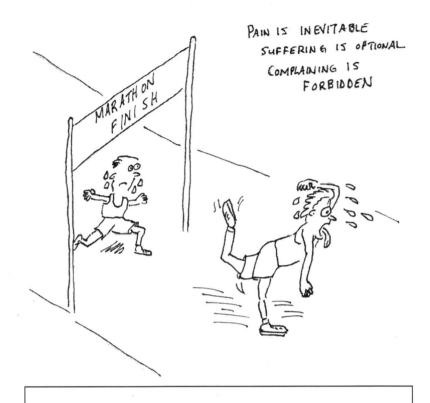

_It's supposed to be hard.
If it was easy,
everyone would do
it!_

MONTH			COURSE	NOTES: temp, wind, pace etc.
day	distance	time		
WEEK		TOTAL		
last wk ytd				
YTD		TOTAL		

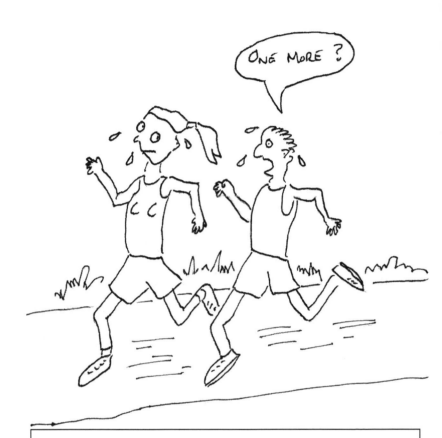

Go the extra mile,
it's never crowded.

MONTH			COURSE	NOTES: temp, wind, pace etc.
day	distance	time		
WEEK		TOTAL		
last wk ytd				
YTD		TOTAL		

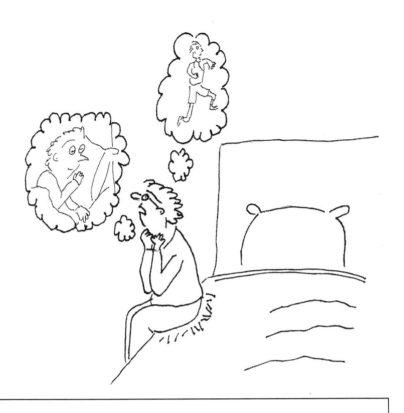

No matter how you feel, get up, dress up, show up and never, ever give up.

MONTH			COURSE	NOTES: temp, wind, pace etc.
day	distance	time		
WEEK		TOTAL		
last wk ytd				
YTD		TOTAL		

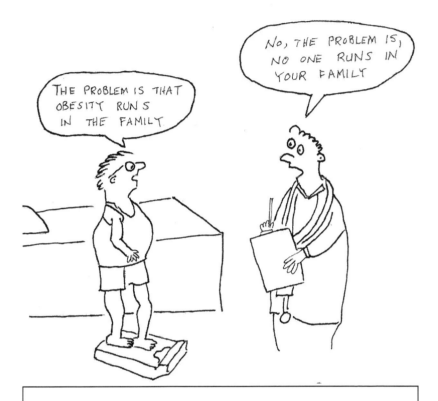

Champions train,
losers complain.

MONTH ___			COURSE	NOTES: temp, wind, pace etc.
day	distance	time		
WEEK ___		TOTAL		
last wk ytd				
YTD		TOTAL		

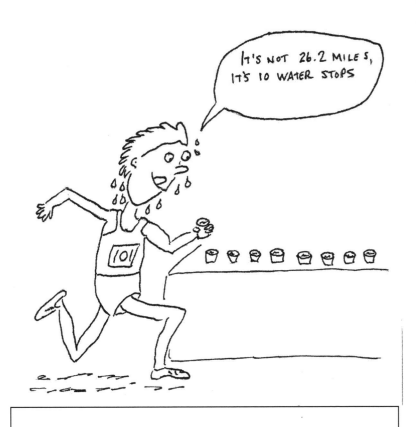

Stay focused with positive thoughts!

MONTH			COURSE	NOTES: temp, wind, pace etc.
day	distance	time		
WEEK		TOTAL		
last wk ytd				
YTD		TOTAL		

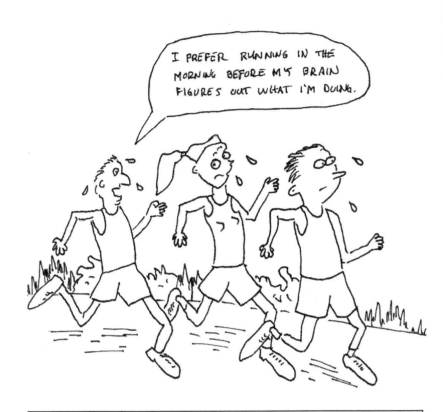

90% of running is half mental.

MONTH	day	distance	time	COURSE	NOTES: temp, wind, pace etc.
WEEK			TOTAL		
last wk ytd					
YTD			TOTAL		

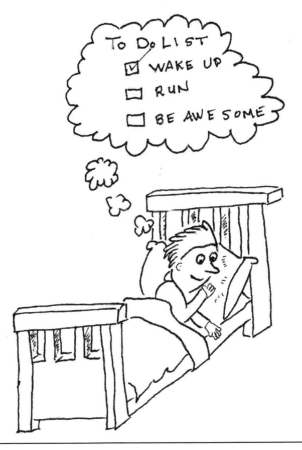

The first
person you have to
inspire every day
is
yourself.

MONTH _____			COURSE	NOTES: temp, wind, pace etc.
day	distance	time		
		TOTAL		
WEEK _____ last wk ytd				
YTD		TOTAL		

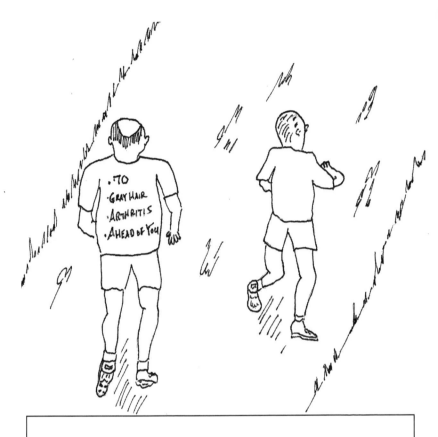

We all need motivation, what's yours?

MONTH			COURSE	NOTES: temp, wind, pace etc.
day	distance	time		
WEEK		TOTAL		
last wk ytd				
YTD		TOTAL		

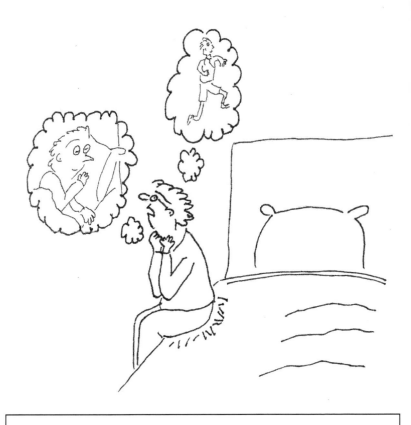

When in doubt, go work out.

MONTH			COURSE	NOTES: temp, wind, pace etc.
day	distance	time		
WEEK		TOTAL		
last wk ytd				
YTD		TOTAL		

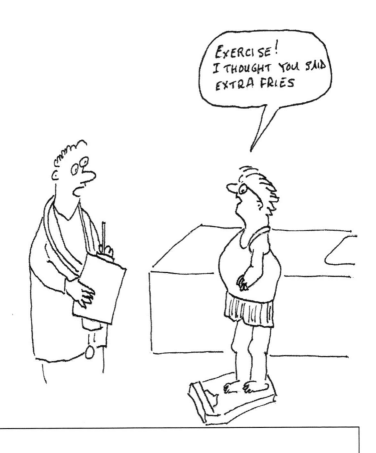

Diet advice: Eat less, exercise more.

MONTH ___			NOTES: temp, wind, pace etc.	COURSE
day	distance	time		
WEEK		TOTAL		
last wk ytd				
YTD		TOTAL		

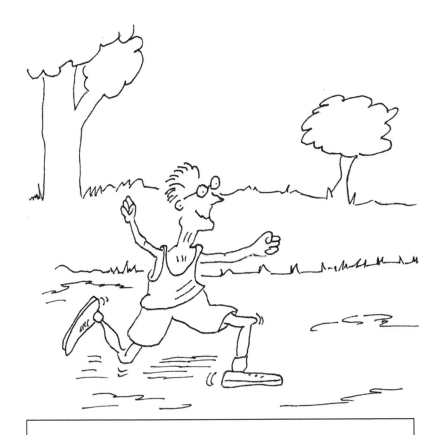

There will be a day when you can no longer do this, today is not that day!

MONTH ___			COURSE	NOTES: temp, wind, pace etc.
day	distance	time		
WEEK		TOTAL		
last wk ytd				
YTD		TOTAL		

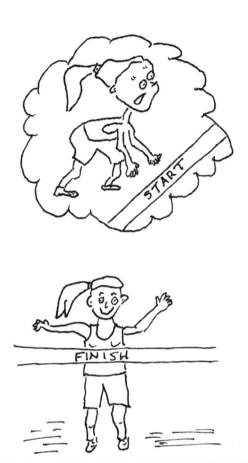

You don't have to
be great to start,
but you do have to
start to be great.

MONTH			COURSE	NOTES: temp, wind, pace etc.
day	distance	time		
		TOTAL		
WEEK last wk ytd				
YTD		TOTAL		

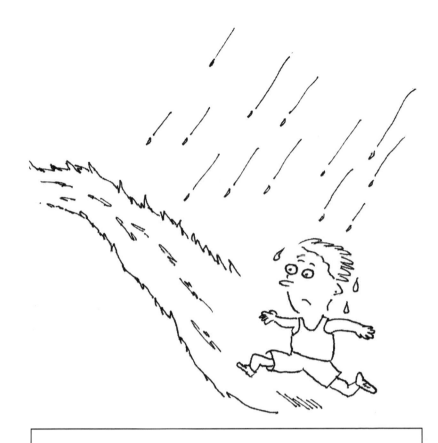

When the going gets tough, the tough run another hill!

MONTH

day	distance	time	COURSE	NOTES: temp, wind, pace etc.
WEEK		TOTAL		
last wk ytd				
YTD		TOTAL		

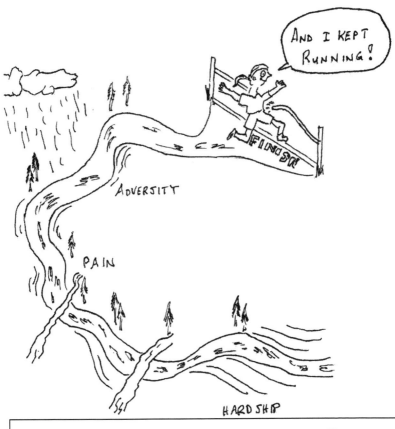

The moment when you want to quit, is the moment when you need to keep pushing.

MONTH			COURSE	NOTES: temp, wind, pace etc.
day	distance	time		
	WEEK	**TOTAL**		
	last wk ytd			
	YTD	**TOTAL**		

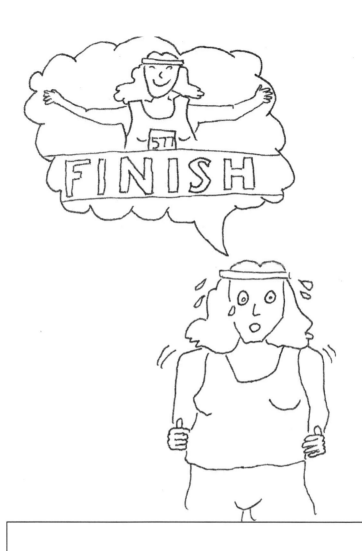

It always seems impossible until it's done.

MONTH____			COURSE	NOTES: temp, wind, pace etc.
day	distance	time		
WEEK		TOTAL		
last wk ytd				
YTD		TOTAL		

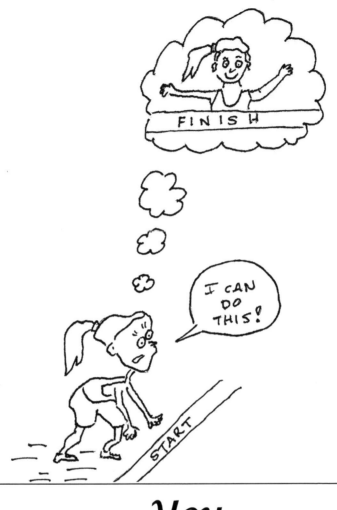

You
believed you could
and you
did!

MONTH			COURSE	NOTES: temp, wind, pace etc.
day	distance	time		
WEEK		TOTAL		
last wk ytd				
YTD		TOTAL		

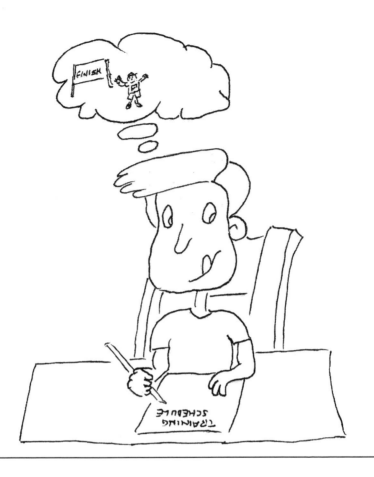

Have a dream, make a plan, go for it.

MONTH			COURSE	NOTES: temp, wind, pace etc.
day	distance	time		
WEEK		TOTAL		
last wk ytd				
YTD		TOTAL		

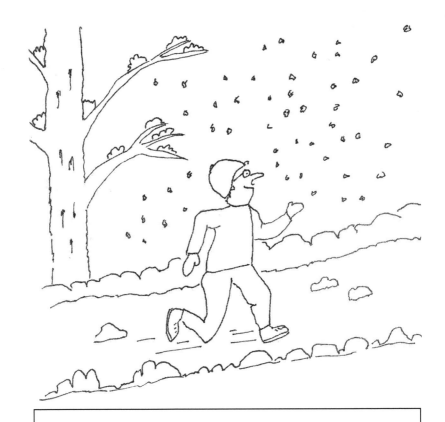

There is no such thing as bad weather, just soft people.

MONTH ___			COURSE	NOTES: temp, wind, pace etc.
day	distance	time		
WEEK		TOTAL		
last wk ytd				
YTD		TOTAL		

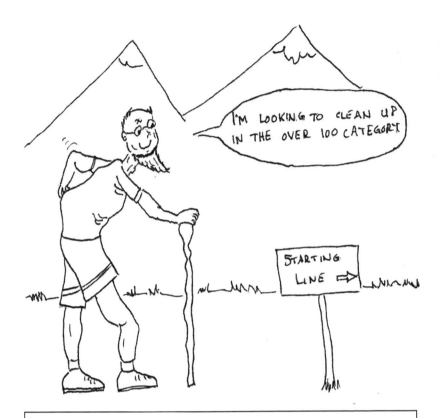

You don't stop run-ning because you get old, you get old because you stop running.

MONTH ___			COURSE	NOTES: temp, wind, pace etc.
day	distance	time		
WEEK		TOTAL		
last wk ytd				
YTD		TOTAL		

ADDENDUM

1. **Why run**

2. **Race history**

3. **Stretching—before and after**

4. **Injuries and treatment**

5. **Injuries and illness Log**

6. **Nutrition tips**

7. **Health tips**

8. **Shoe history**

9. **Sample training plan for beginners**

10. **Running Terms**

11. **Things runners do every day**

12. **Notes and comments**

Why Run?

Well, there are as many reasons as there are runners.

1. To compete. Running is an activity that allows anyone, regardless of age, to compete against others in the same age bracket from preteens to octogenarians.
2. To achieve a PR (Personal Record). No matter the age or gender, it's always nice to know that you can do better.
3. To relieve stress. Worries about job, family, current events can take their toll, running is a great way to put things back in perspective.
4. To stay fit. Running is one of the best and most efficient ways to maintain cardiovascular health.

5. To socialize. Running is a great way to meet new people all with the same interest but with every conceivable background.

6. To save money. No need for expensive club dues, no need for expensive equipment. Other than a good pair of running shoes all you need is the open road.

7. To save time. No need to drive to the gym or club, no need to schedule a time, just lace up and get out the front door any time of day or night.

8. To spend time with the family. Running is a sport for all ages. Get the spouse, the kids, other family members and go for a run together. You'll make memories to last a lifetime.

JUST DO IT! (Nike slogan)

Lace up, dress up, buck up

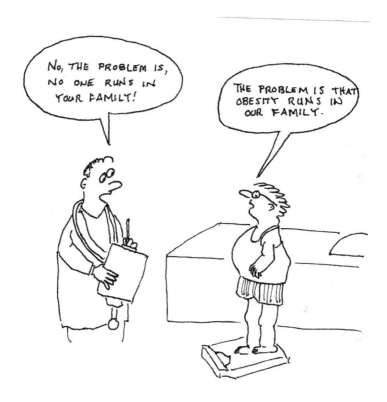

RACE HISTORY

Hey, I get it, not everyone likes to race, you'd rather it's just you and the open road, but, think of it, how else are you going to get T-shirts?

It's also a great way to really determine how good a shape you are really in and charity races are a great way for you to support your favorite charity(ies).

On the following pages you can record up to six races that you've run in over the year. It's a great way to look back at the highlights of your year and, if you run the same races year after year, it's a great way to recall those memorable (and maybe not so memorable) events from the years past.

Race name:_____

Town:_____

Distance:_____

Time:_____

Course type:_____

Your place (overall):_____

Age-group place:_____

Comments:_____

_____

_____

_____

━━━━━━━━━━━━━━━━━━━━━━━━━━━

Race name:_____

Town:_____

Distance:_____

Time:_____

Course type:_____

Your place (overall):_____

Age-group place:_____

Comments:_____

_____

_____

_____

Race name:_____

Town:_____

Distance:_____

Time:_____

Course type:_____

Your place (overall):_____

Age-group place:_____

Comments:_____

_____

_____

_____

Race name:_____

Town:_____

Distance:_____

Time:_____

Course type:_____

Your place (overall):_____

Age-group place:_____

Comments:_____

_____

_____

_____

Race name:_____

Town:_____

Distance:_____

Time:_____

Course type:_____

Your place (overall):_____

Age-group place:_____

Comments:_____

_____

_____

_____

━━━━━━━━━━━━━━━━━━━━━━━━━━

Race name:_____

Town:_____

Distance:_____

Time:_____

Course type:_____

Your place (overall):_____

Age-group place:_____

Comments:_____

_____

_____

_____

Stretching

This topic gets a lot of discussion and debate currently. When should I stretch, how much, how long etc.

Some say no stretching before hand is necessary, just walk for a few minutes and jog slowly before running. Others advocate stretching before and after.

Personally, every run that I've attended, runners are doing all of the above. My recommendation? Do whatever works for you. If you want to stretch prior to your run, do so but ease into each stretch and do it slowly so you feel comfortable.

Stretch after each run to maintain your flexibility and help to eliminate any tightness.

I've provided a few suggestion here for before and after just to get you started and then you can improvise from there.

Warm Up Stretching
Dynamic

1. Hip Circles:

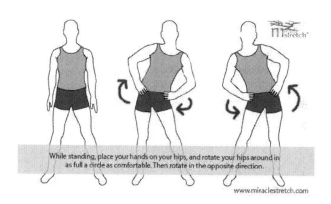

While standing, place your hands on your hips, and rotate your hips around in as full a circle as comfortable. Then rotate in the opposite direction.

www.miraclestretch.com

2. Walking Lunges:

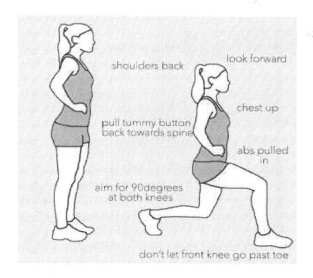

shoulders back

look forward

chest up

pull tummy button back towards spine

abs pulled in

aim for 90degrees at both knees

don't let front knee go past toe

Warm Up Stretching
Dynamic

3. Butt Kicks:

Butt kicks

How
- Start jogging in place. Begin to quickly bring your heel up toward your buttock.

Benefits
- Butt kicks are one of the best ways to warm up your leg muscles and increase your circulation and core body temperature. If you're a runner, you may notice that butt kicks improve your running posture and stride, too.

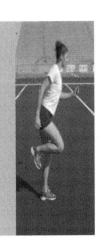

4. Leg Swing:

Forward-and-Back Leg Swings

1. Stand tall and hold on to a sturdy object with your left hand. Brace your core.
2. Keeping your right knee straight, swing your right leg forward as high as you comfortably can.
3. Swing your right leg backward as far as you can. That's one rep. Swing back and forth continuously.
4. Complete all your reps, then do the same with your left leg.

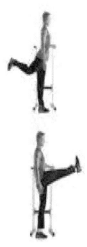

Warm Up Stretching
Dynamic

5. Leg Swing:

Lateral Leg Swing

1. Stand tall.
2. Allow the leg to be "loose" in the hip socket.
3. Swing one leg front to back 10x.
4. Repeat on other leg.
5. Then swing leg laterally, out and across the midline of the body, 10x each side.

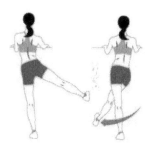

6. High Knees:

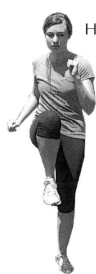

High Knees

Quickly lift one leg toward your chest (keeping abs tight...focus on using your core to raise your leg). Switch legs as fast as you can while maintaining control of your movement. Aim to raise your knees to hip height each time.

Stretching
Post Run

1. Calf stretch:

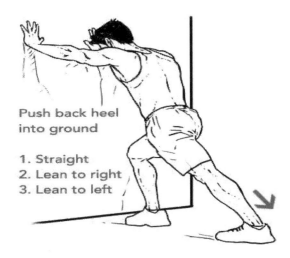

Push back heel
into ground

1. Straight
2. Lean to right
3. Lean to left

2. Hamstrings:

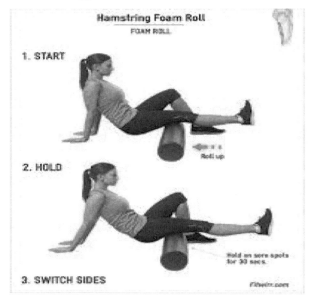

Hamstring Foam Roll

FOAM ROLL

1. START

Roll up

2. HOLD

Hold on sore spots
for 30 secs.

3. SWITCH SIDES

Fitwirx.com

Stretching
Post Run

3. Groin stretch:

Groin Stretch
Standing

Position

Lunge slowly to the left while keeping the right leg straight, the right foot facing straight ahead and entirely on the floor.

Action

Lean over the left leg while stretching the right groin muscles. Hold this position for 10-15 seconds. Repeat with the opposite leg.

Groin Stretch
Seated

Position

Sit on the ground with the soles together. Place the hands on or near the feet.

Action

Bend forward from the hips, keeping the head up. Hold this position for 10-15 seconds.

4. Hip Stretch:

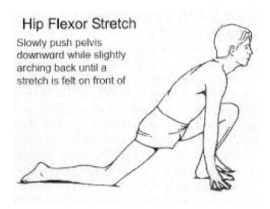

Hip Flexor Stretch

Slowly push pelvis downward while slightly arching back until a stretch is felt on front of

5. Back Stretch

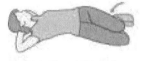

NB: Upper knee should be directly above lower knee.

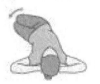

Back stretch

Lie on your back, hands above your head. Bend your knees and roll them slowly to one side, keeping your feet on the floor. Hold for 10 seconds. Repeat 3 times on each side.

Injuries and Treatment

1. Achilles Tendinitis:

A dull or sharp pain along the Achilles tendon, usually close to the heel. Can be caused by excessive hill running, overtraining, lack of warm up or improper foot wear. Best treatment is to cut down on running, massage frequently, ice, take aspirin.

2. Blisters:

Blisters are caused by friction on the skin creating irritation and a body reaction creating the blister. Shoes may be too tight, too loose, feet are wet, socks are slipping etc. Treatment is cleaning the area with alcohol, lancing with a sterile needle and covering with a gauze pad and keeping the foot dry until healing has occurred. Lubricant (petroleum jelly) may help reoccurrence.

3. Iliotibial Band Syndrome (IBS):

This is a pain occurring on the outside of the knee caused by the ligament rubbing against the femur. It can be caused by worn out shoes, speeding up workouts too quickly, downhill workouts or running on banked circuits. Best treatment is to stop running, cross train, regular stretching and icing.

4. Plantar Fasciitis:

This pain occurs at the base of the heel. It may feel like you've stepped on a stone but the pain won't go away. If you have high arches or flat feet you may be susceptible. Lack of stretching, worn out shoes may be the cause. Reduce your running, stretch , ice the area, roll a ball under your foot 3 times per day.

Injuries and Treatment

3. Shin splints:

Pain occurring on either side of the shin, halfway down or all along the shin, tendinitis of the lower leg. Usually the result of too much too soon, especially with beginning runners. Also aggravated by running on hard surfaces (concrete) or running stairs (concrete) Cut down on your running, ice the shins frequently, consider wrapping your legs until condition goes away.

4. Runners Knee:

One of the more common problems experienced by runners. It can be caused by weak quads, tight hamstring and calf muscles, running on uneven surfaces or hills. Best treatment is to reduce running, stay on flat, softer (trail) surfaces, consider orthotics.

Injuries and Treatment

5. Other common Issues:

- <u>Athletes Foot</u>—Try isopropyl alcohol spray to dry your skin
- <u>Cramps or stitches</u>-stabbing pain just below the rib cage. Try expanding your diaphragm by breathing from your belly. Strengthen your abs.
- <u>Diarrhea</u>-Use the bathroom before you run, cut back on fiber, drink more water, cut back on dairy products.

NOTE: If any injury does not respond to self treatment in a short period of time DON'T attempt to "gut it out". See a medical professional for proper treatment so the condition doesn't become a problem that could sideline you permanently.

Injuries/Illness Log

Injury/Illness_____

Date_____

Length of recuperation_____

Cause_____

_____

Treatment_____

_____

Comments_____

_____

Injury/Illness_____

Date_____

Length of recuperation_____

Cause_____

_____

Treatment_____

_____

Comments_____

_____

Injuries/Illness Log

Injury/Illness_____

Date_____

Length of recuperation_____

Cause_____

_____

Treatment_____

_____

Comments_____

_____

_____

Injury/Illness_____

Date_____

Length of recuperation_____

Cause_____

_____

Treatment_____

_____

Comments_____

_____

Nutrition Tips
(excerpted from Runners World Training Guide)

1. How many calories a day do you need? Here's a way to estimate:
- Multiply your goal weight by 10
- Add to that 20% if you ride a desk, 50% if you're reasonably active and 70% if you're on your feet all day.
- Add the calories burned during your workout (see formula below)
- Reduce the total by 15%

The calculated figure is an estimate of the calories you require daily to achieve/maintain your goal weight and be able to go about your daily activities and exercise routines

Formula for calculating calories burned during a workout:
<u>Distance run X weight X 0.76 factor = calories burned</u>

Nutrition Tips
(excerpted from Runners World Training Guide)

1. Eat real foods. Fish, chicken, vegetables, whole grains, low fat dairy, fruits, nuts provide plenty of nutritional value. Stay away from fast foods and highly processed foods.
2. You need carbohydrates so consider grains (pasta), fruits and vegetables. Again, the less processed the better.
3. Stay hydrated but cut down on fruit drinks, stay away from soda and have a cup of coffee or tea in place of that mocha. After a workout consider a sports drink to replace fluids and electrolytes. During the rest of the day drink water between meals
4. Consider keeping track of your meals/eating habits. Are you snacking too much?
5. Indulge occasionally!

Nutrition Tips
(excerpted from Runners World Training Guide)

Lose weight, improve nutrition with these substitutions:

1. Olive oil vs creamy dressing—save 90 calories
2. Organic fat free milk vs 2% - save 30 calories
3. Club soda with fruit juice vs fruit drinks—save 50 calories
4. Whole grain bread versus white bread—increased fiber
5. Dark beer vs light beer—more anti-oxidants.
6. Roasted chicken vs deli meats—reduced sodium.
7. Radishes, peppers, snow peas vs celery—more nutrients
8. Low carb tortillas vs white flour tortillas—save 60 calories
9. Baby greens vs iceberg lettuce—added carotenes

Nutrition Tips
(post run only?

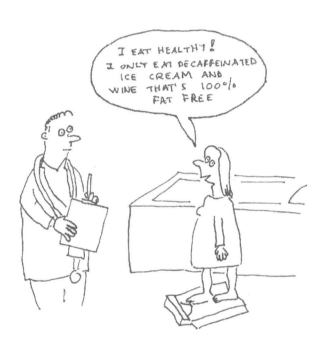

Health Tips

1. If you are planning to start a running program, good for you! Check with your doctor to ensure there are no underlining concerns.
2. Get a good pair of running shoes! Don't scrimp, go to a store dedicated to runners to get the right fit and style for you.
3. Alternate running shoes every other day to allow for them to dry out.
4. Warm up before hand with a short walk, cool down afterward with stretches and a walk.
5. Outside in the summer? Wear a sunscreen (SPF 15 or higher) and a hat.
6. Cut down on salt but do drink a sports drink to replenish electrolytes.

Health Tips

7. Winter running? If you're warm starting out you're overdressed. Skip the heavy jacket and go with a shell, long sleeve technical shirt and t-shirt instead.

8. Headset—Don't wear them when running outside, it's just plain not safe!

9. Hot outside? Slow down, stay hydrated, consider running in the early hours when it's cooler.

10. Running at night or sundown? Wear a reflective vest and take/wear a light at all times. Stay off the roads, drivers may not see you.

11. Consider cross training on those off days; swimming, bicycling, rowing, trail walking, skiing, strength training.

12. RELAX, have fun. The benefits are many.

Shoe History

Shoe Brand:_____

Model:_____

Size:_____**Price:**_____

Where purchased:_____

_____

Date purchased:_____

Date discarded:_____

Comments:_____

_____

_____

_____

Shoe Brand:_____

Model:_____

Size: _____**Price:**_____

Where purchased:_____

_____

Date purchased:_____

Date discarded:_____

Comments:_____

_____

_____

_____

Training Plan

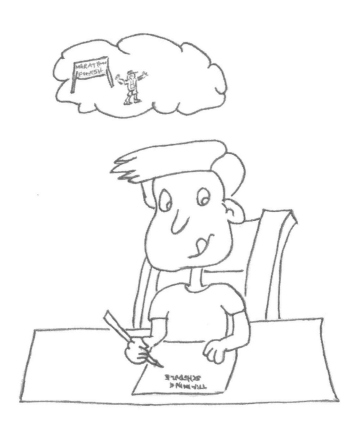

Have a dream, make a plan, go for it!

Sample Training Plan
for beginners

1. Before you begin check with your health professional to be sure you are ready for aerobic activity.
2. Go to a local running store and get a good pair of running shoes. Let a trained professional fit you in the correct shoe for your size, gait and type of running.
3. Select a running venue. It could be a local park, a local trail or local running club. Anyplace you feel comfortable.
4. Pick a running partner if at all possible, a good friend, a spouse of one of your children who also wants to start. If you both make a commitment you'll feel compelled to get out the door.
5. Finally, pick a time of day that works best for you. Mornings are most common but whatever works.

Sample Training Plan Program

NOTE: At any time you can modify this program to meet your needs, just remember not to overdo it and get burnt out.

- **1st & 2nd weeks: Walk actively for 30 minutes (get your heart rate up) at least 3 times per week.**

- **3rd & 4th weeks: Walk for 9 minutes, run for 1 minute comfortably.**

- **5th & 6th weeks: Walk 8 minutes, run 2 minutes.**

- **7th & 8th weeks: Walk 7, run 3.**

- **9th & 10 weeks : Walk 6, run 4.**

- **11th & 12th weeks: Walk 5, run 5.**

Sample Training Plan Program

At this point you should be able to decide if you want to stay with the 2 week plan or move up to a 1 week plan.

- 13th week: Walk 4, run 6

- 14th week: Walk 3, run 7

- 15th week: walk 2, run 8

- 16th week: walk 1, run 9

Sign up for a Local 5K run in 2 weeks!

- 17th & 18th weeks run 30 minutes at least 3 times each week

Take a rest day before the race.

Have fun, enjoy the race,

Running Terms

Pace: Speed at which you are running. Expressed in minutes/mile or kilometer.

Interval training: A training day with alternate periods of speed work and recovery periods of low intensity.

Fartlek: A Swedish term meaning "Speed Play". In running, any unstructured workout perhaps through fields and forested trails.

5K: Five Kilometers (3.1 miles). A perfect race distance for beginners and recreational runners.

10K: Ten Kilometers (6.2 miles). Perfect race for intermediate runners moving up to the next level of competition.

Half Marathon: 13.1 miles. Second to the last step before a full marathon.

Full Marathon: 26.2 miles. You've arrived. This should be on everyone's bucket list.

Running Terms

Ultras (or Ultra Marathons): Any distance beyond a marathon. 50 K, 50 miles, 100 miles et al.

PR: Personal Record or PB, Personal Best.

Bib: Printed square that each runner pins on preferably to the front of their racing shirt. Their unique identifier.

Chip: Computerized disk attached within bib of to a running shoe to track exact run time. Activated on passing electronic mat at start and stops when runner crosses finish.

Negative Splits: Running the second half of a race faster than the first half.

Bandit: Someone who is running a race without registering and paying and is unofficial.

Running Terms

Repeats: Fast segments of a workout with recovery periods in between. Used to build speed.

Tempo runs: Runs that are comfortable hard. Good for building endurance.

10% rule: Maximum suggested % increase in distance over previous workout routine. 5% suggested for older runners.

DNF: Did Not Finish.

Masters Runner: An athlete over 40 years of age.

Endorphins: Causal factor in "runners high". A feeling of elation after a hard run and workout.

Hill Repeats: Running up a hill at race pace and trotting back down for a number of repeats. Build speed and strength.

Things runners do every day

1. They keep a running log. Tracking your daily activity plus results from your races is a great motivation tool.

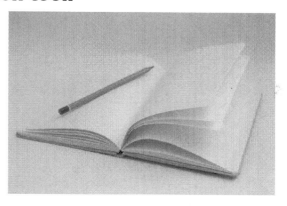

2. They schedule their runs. Like anything else in their day, it becomes "to do" task.

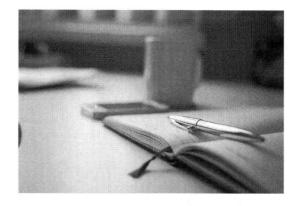

Things runners do every day

3. They eat healthy. They are sure to eat a healthy meal and stay hydrated after every run.

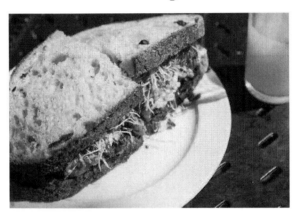

4. They take time to rest and recover.

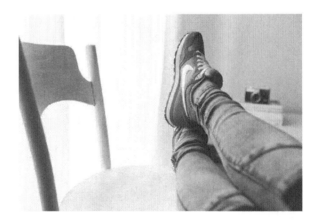

Things runners do every day

5. They keep track of their shoes. 400 to 500 miles and it's probably time for a new pair.

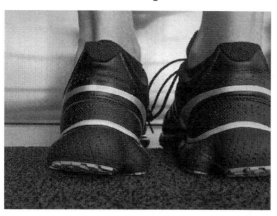

6. They cross train. Yoga, bicycling, swimming are ways to keep fresh while still maintaining fitness

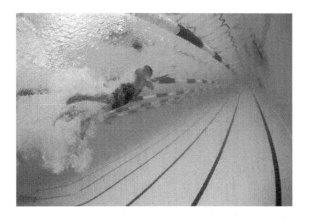

Notes & Comments

_____

_____

_____

_____

_____

_____

_____

_____

_____

_____

_____

_____

_____

_____

_____

_____

_____

_____

_____

_____

—

Notes & Comments

82609751R00089

Made in the USA
Columbia, SC
18 December 2017